HERBAL MEDICINE

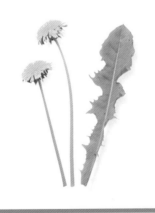

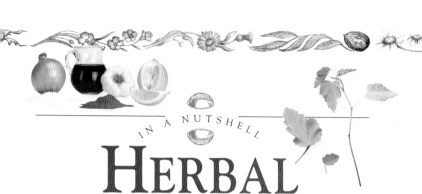

IN A NUTSHELL

HERBAL
MEDICINE
A STEP-BY-STEP
GUIDE

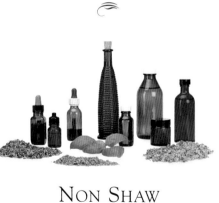

NON SHAW

ELEMENT

SHAFTESBURY, DORSET • BOSTON, MASSACHUSETTS • MELBOURNE, VICTORIA

© Element Books Limited 1998

First published in
Great Britain in 1998 by
ELEMENT BOOKS LIMITED
Shaftesbury, Dorset, SP7 9BP

Published in the USA in 1998 by
ELEMENT BOOKS INC
160 North Washington Street, Boston,
Massachusetts 02114

Published in Australia in 1998 by
ELEMENT BOOKS LIMITED
and distributed by Penguin Australia Ltd,
487 Maroondah Highway, Ringwood,
Victoria 3134

Reprinted September 1998

NOTE FROM THE PUBLISHER
Any information given in this
book is not intended to be
taken as a replacement for
medical advice. Any
person with a
condition requiring
medical attention
should consult a
qualified practitioner or
therapist.

ISBN 1 86204 196 2

Printed ad bound in
Italy by
Graphicom

Designed and created with
The Bridgewater Book Company Ltd

ELEMENT BOOKS LIMITED
Managing Editor Miranda Spicer
Senior Commissioning Editor Caro Ness
Production Manager Susan Sutterby
Production Controller Fiona Harrison
Project Editor Katie Worrall

THE BRIDGEWATER BOOK COMPANY LTD
Art Director Terry Jeavons
Designer Glyn Bridgewater
Page layout Glyn Bridgewater
Managing Editor Anne Townley
Project Manager Fiona Corbridge
Picture Research Lynda Marshall
Three-dimensional models Mark Jamieson
Photography Ian Parsons
Illustrations Andrew Kulman

British Library Cataloguing in
Publication data available

Library of Congress Cataloging
in Publication data available

The publishers wish to thank the
following for the use of pictures:
Bridgeman Art Library: 6T, 6B,
7, 8T; Garden Picture Library:
6L, 17B, 21T, 22T, 24R, 27,
29C, 31TR, 37T, 38T, 41TL

Special thanks go to:
Lily Adams, Natasha Gray,
Julia Holden, Natalie Jerome,
Darren Law, Anna Rawson,
Lesley and Sammy Thomas
for help with
photography

Contents

What is herbal medicine?

HERBAL MEDICINE IS THE USE *of plants as remedies to restore health. Many orthodox drugs originated from plant extracts, but the difference between orthodox and herbal medicine is that herbalists believe the whole plant makes a more balanced medicine than purified extracts.*

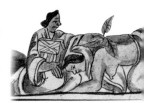

ABOVE: *An Aztec woman using herbs after childbirth.*

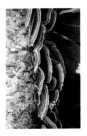

ABOVE: *Birch fungus has been used since the Stone Age. It disinfects wounds.*

Herbalism is the oldest complementary therapy. In prehistoric times, when people hunted and gathered plants, there was little difference between food and medicine. Plants were picked, as available, to meet needs. Some needs recurred day after day, for example, the need for energy, carbohydrates, and protein. Other needs, for example a styptic antiseptic for a wound or an astringent for diarrhea, only cropped up occasionally. As the culture developed, the sustaining plants needed every day were cultivated by farmers. The knowledge of occasional "healing and rebalancing" plants was passed

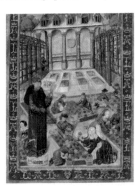

ABOVE: *A French 15th-century manuscript depicting a garden of medicinal plants.*

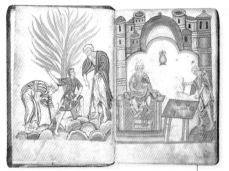

Books containing herbal lore, often richly illustrated, have been produced for centuries.

to a particular person or family. Thus wise women, healers, shamans, and eventually herbalists and doctors, came into existence. They were knowledge-holders, ready to share their specialized skill at times of need.

Herbalism has always been divided into two areas: home remedies and professional remedies. Home remedies are suitable for first aid, for treating minor complaints, and for the home care of sick people. Professional remedies are more specialized, often using stronger and rarer herbs, and learned skills of diagnosis and treatment.

There is plenty of historical evidence revealing the use of herbs. The Stone Age "iceman"

found frozen in the Austrian alps some years ago carried with him a first-aid kit of two small pieces of birch fungus. Birch fungus is still used to stop bleeding and disinfect wounds. St Hildegard, an 11th-century Swiss abbess, knew of six different types of healing fungus, maintained a large garden of medicinal herbs, and even imported herbs from the Indies. Sick people who had exhausted their homely reserves would visit her to obtain rare herbs or receive specialized treatments.

MEDICAL HERBALISM

Medical herbalism is the use of plants as medicines to restore and maintain health by keeping the body in balance. It relies on the curative qualities of specific plants, flowers, trees, and herbs to stimulate our own healing system and restore health. Like most holistic practitioners, herbalists believe that we all possess healing energy, which they call the vital force. This vital force works constantly to maintain the health of the whole person – physical, mental, and emotional.

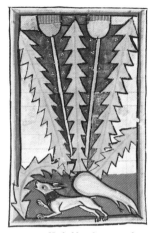

ABOVE: *Herbal lore has crossed international boundaries. This medicinal plant comes from a Latin translation of a Greek herbal.*

Home treatment reached its highest point with the ladies of the manor in England in the 17th and 18th centuries. A close community of 100 or so people would have lived and worked on the manor house estate. Their needs were mostly provided for by what they could grow for themselves, with the addition of the occasional purchase of exotics such as sugar and raisins. The ladies kept their recipes in "still room books," which included cures for wounds and fevers, methods for dyeing, for making soap, and for preserving fruit. The medicines were part of everyday life. Doctors would be sent for only in extreme circumstances.

One well-known doctor was John Hall, who was married to William Shakespeare's daughter and was famous for his cure for scurvy, which contained plenty of fresh watercress juice, amongst other herbs.

PLANTS IN OUR LIVES

Plants are used to enrich all aspects of our lives. We depend on them for things ranging from the dye in our cloth to the oxygen in the air. People have depended on plants since the earliest times. Isolated communities had to be totally self-sufficient. For example, the Pilgrim Fathers took herbs and medicinal plants with them to America. Plantain was called "Englishman's foot" by the natives, as they noticed that it sprang up everywhere the settlers went.

PLANTAIN

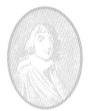

ABOVE: *Nicholas Culpeper was a famous 16th-century herbalist who wrote a famous book called* The Complete Herbal.

Many of the great herbals were written 300 years ago – by herbalists such as Culpeper, Gerard, Coles, and Turner – but they are still useful today. The herbs work, although why and how is poorly understood and most plant stratagems have not yet been explored. Modern science is vindicating traditional herbal practices, such as putting moldy bread on to a wound (primitive penicillin), or drinking mare's urine for infertility (today some hormone replacement therapy products are made from mare's urine). Tradition, personal experience, an open mind, and common sense make up the home herbalist's guide.

There is a whole area in which plants can be used, not as sustaining food, or even as medicines, but in between, as strengthening tonics and preventatives to maintain optimum well-being. This is the realm of this little book.

SOME USES OF HERBS

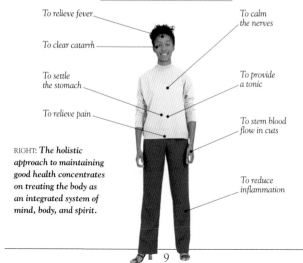

To relieve fever

To clear catarrh

To settle the stomach

To relieve pain

To calm the nerves

To provide a tonic

To stem blood flow in cuts

To reduce inflammation

RIGHT: *The holistic approach to maintaining good health concentrates on treating the body as an integrated system of mind, body, and spirit.*

How herbs work

HERBAL REMEDIES ALLOW US *to care for ourselves and each other using the resources of the planet as directly as possible – they are a safe and simple connection.*

ABOVE: **Herbal methods of treatment are seen to be more in tune with the conservation of the environment.**

Many people have moved toward "natural" remedies in response to the tragic results and side-effects of some drugs, and as a backlash against the huge multinational profit-orientated drug companies. Herbs are perceived to be a purer, safer alternative, and an intimate and renewable resource. But it is important to exercise caution, because herbs are profoundly powerful tools of healing. They should always be used in moderation.

BELOW: **This model shows the molecular structure of citric acid, which is found in citrus fruits.**

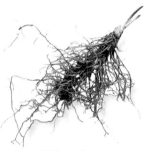

ABOVE: **Golden seal root contains alkaloids, essential oil traces, resin, and fatty oil. It is good for catarrh and digestive problems.**

ORGANIC HERBS

It is important to remember that herbs can be abused before you buy them – for example, grown as a mono crop with the aid of pesticides, and irradiated. If you care about such issues, buy organic herbs and ask about the conditions of their growth, picking, transportation, packaging, and storage.

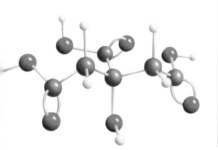

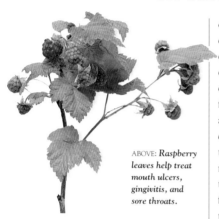

ABOVE: *Raspberry leaves help treat mouth ulcers, gingivitis, and sore throats.*

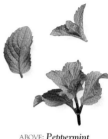

ABOVE: *Peppermint is a very versatile herb. It is an excellent stomach relaxant.*

container, then sit down for a quarter of an hour and experience its full effects, from the first sniff of steam acting as a decongestant, to the soothing, relaxing warmth in the stomach after five minutes, and the general feeling of improved well-being and mental clarity spreading out after ten. A relaxing mild stimulant!

Orthodox medicine works by aiming one purified ingredient at a specific site, almost like a "magic bullet." Herbs work by strengthening the body so that it is more able to cope. They contain an amalgam of ingredients which work together, using complex mechanisms to buffer and support. Consider the many actions of peppermint. It is a warming digestive, anti-spasmodic, mild stimulant, and decongestant. It clears gas, relaxes the intestines, relieves colic, and lifts the spirits. These might sound contradictory, but to understand, make yourself a strong cup of peppermint tea. Brew it properly in a closed

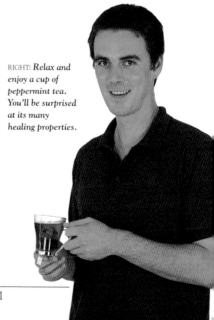

RIGHT: *Relax and enjoy a cup of peppermint tea. You'll be surprised at its many healing properties.*

Using herbs

WILLOW BARK

HERBS CAN BE USED IN *a great variety of ways – in teas, infusions, decoctions, syrups, oils, ointments, and compresses to name but a few. The kind of treatment used depends both on the herb in question and the ailment.*

ABOVE:
Chamomile is a gentle herb suitable for children. Chamomile tea aids digestion.

HERBAL TEAS OR INFUSIONS

Infusing herb in hot water is the most pleasant and effective method of taking many of them. The human body has an affinity for water, and infusions can be tolerated by children and those with weakened systems.

Infusions are most suitable for leaves or flowers, such as yarrow or chamomile. Seeds and roots may be used in infusions but they are left to brew for twice as long.

MAKING AN INFUSION

☞ Use 1 teaspoon of dried herb (or 2 of chopped, fresh herb) to 1 cup of water. Use a closed container. Small teapots that have a built-in strainer are ideal. Tea bags can be used for general drinking purposes but freshly bought loose herbs are better for medicinal use.

☞ Dose: 3 cups a day for long-term use. Up to 6 cups a day for acute conditions such as flu.
☞ Herbs are complex remedies: take time to get all the effects. Let the steam clear your head, notice the effect in the stomach, and then the general feeling in the body 10 minutes after drinking.

1 *Pour boiling water on to the herbs.*

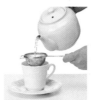

2 *After 5 minutes, pour, strain, and drink.*

DECOCTIONS

These are suitable for roots, barks, and seeds, such as dandelion root and willow bark. Use 1oz (25g) of herb to 1 pint (500ml) of water. Bring to the boil, and simmer for 10 minutes and strain. Decoctions may be kept in the fridge for a few days.

☞ Dose: ½ cup 3–6 times daily.

MAKING A DECOCTION

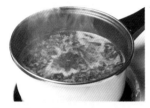

1 Use a glass, ceramic or enamelled pan. Cover, and simmer herbs for 10 minutes.

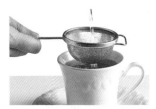

2 Strain the tea while it is hot. Use the decoction within a few days.

SYRUPS

These can be made from decoctions. First make your decoction then slowly reduce it, over a low heat, to one eighth of its volume. Measure. Add 2lb (1kg) of sugar to every 1 pint (500ml) of liquid. Return to a low heat and stir until the sugar dissolves. Store in sterilized bottles in a cool place. Syrups will keep for some months.

☞ Dose: 1 dessertspoonful 3–6 times daily.

TREATING CHILDREN

Use half doses for children over 7 and quarter doses for children between 5 and 7. For infants, use only a teaspoonful or follow the instructions of your herbalist.

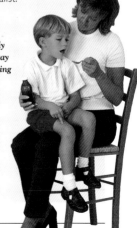

RIGHT:
Syrups are an especially palatable way of encouraging children to take herbal remedies.

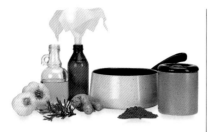

ABOVE: *Equipment for making infused oils: pan, container, bottles, strainer, oil and herbs.*

INFUSED OILS

These are suitable for massage, chest rubs, etc. Find a small pottery or stainless steel container with a good lid and a pan large enough for it to stand in with plenty of room to spare. Chop enough fresh herb to fill the container twice. Put half the herb into the container and pour on enough olive or sunflower oil to cover. Put the lid on and stand the container in the pan. Pour water into the pan to come half-way up the container. Place on the stove and bring the water to the boil. Simmer for 2 hours. Take care not to let the water boil away. Allow to cool. Strain off the oil and reserve it. Put the rest of the herb into the container, pour on the reserved oil, and repeat the procedure. This method produces a double-strength oil which will keep for some months. Infusing herbs in hot oil allows the release of essential oils.

OINTMENTS AND SALVES

These can be made from infused oils by adding some beeswax to 2 teaspoonfuls (10ml) of infused oil. Grate the beeswax and melt it into the oil over a low heat. Then pour the ointment directly into small jars.

ABOVE: *Herbal ointments are easy to make yourself by adding beeswax to infused oil.*

MASSAGE OILS

All infused oils are warming and nourishing for the skin, and make bases for massage oils. Pure essential oils, extracted from various parts of a plant, can also be made into massage oils but should never be used neat on the skin. Essential oils can be bought at good health shops. Massage oils can also be made using essential oils: add 20–30 drops of essential oil to 2fl oz (50ml) of carrier oil. Shake well and bottle. Do not exceed this strength. Suitable carrier oils include almond oil and herbal-infused oils.

OTHER TREATMENTS WITH HERBS

Infusions and decoctions can be used locally in a number of different ways.

↝ **Wash** – use tea or decoction directly on the skin. Pat dry.

↝ **Soak** – use warm tea at half strength. For stiff hands, soak hands for 15 minutes. For cold feet and poor circulation, soak feet for 10 minutes in a foot bath using a pinch of cayenne.

↝ **Gargle** – gargle for 2 minutes with tea, frequently.

↝ **Douche** – use tepid, half-strength tea, once or twice a day.

↝ **Fomentation** – this is a warm compress. Dip cloth in hot tea, wring, and apply. For warming cold joints.

↝ **Compress** – use cold. Dip cloth in cold tea, wring, and apply. Tea bags can be used as fomentation and compresses. Make sure they are the correct temperature before applying them.

RIGHT: *Applying a calendula compress to relieve the pain of a minor burn. Calendula is good for any skin inflammation.*

Many other preparations – tablets, capsules, creams, tinctures – can be bought ready-made. Follow the instructions on the packet. More detailed instructions can be found in the Materia Medica section starting on page 20.

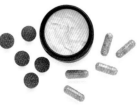

RIGHT: *You can find many pre-prepared treatments at your local herbal pharmacy or health food store.*

Visiting a practitioner

PROFESSIONAL CONSULTANT *medical herbalists are often trained in orthodox diagnosis and can advise on treatment of ailments for which you might usually consult a general physician.*

Accredited members of organizations such as the National Institute of Medical Herbalists in the UK, have undergone four years of study and two years of supervision. They will understand all the various indications and contra-indications of herbs, and any problems which may arise from taking orthodox drugs. A list of organizations which keep a register of qualified practitioners is given at the back of this book.

WHICH CONDITIONS CAN BE TREATED?

Many people only consider consulting a professional herbalist as a last resort, when everything else has failed. For example, herbalists see many

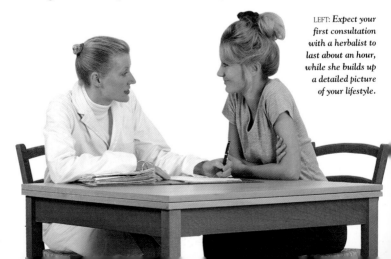

LEFT: *Expect your first consultation with a herbalist to last about an hour, while she builds up a detailed picture of your lifestyle.*

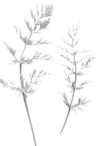

RIGHT: *Caraway is used to treat a range of symptoms, including colic, flatulence, asthma, and period pain.*

people with chronic conditions such as arthritis, chronic fatigue syndrome (ME), and asthma. But not surprisingly, herbalism is best used as a simple first resort. Herbalism can prevent the condition worsening, strengthen the body, and act as a preventative. A herbalist is not simply looking for a "cure," but for an overall improvement in well-being. Professional herbalism can either suggest a comprehensive alternative for those who do not wish to use drugs, or it can offer a system complementary to a course of conventional treatment.

WHAT TO EXPECT

A consultation will take about an hour and cover all aspects of your health, diet, exercise, and lifestyle. Your herbalist will take a "holistic" view, which means taking into consideration everything that affects your health on a physical, mental, and spiritual level.

Your herbalist will want to know how you feel and will note your appearance. There may also be a physical examination.

Many of the herbs prescribed will be familiar to you but some will be unknown. After a consultation a herbalist is able to prescribe herbs which are limited by law and not freely available over the counter to the general public. For example, *Datura stramonium* may be included in an inhalant, to relax the chest during an episode of asthma, or *Convallaria majalis* (lily of the valley) may be used for heart failure. These herbs are powerful and effective, and must only be taken under professional guidance.

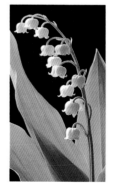

RIGHT: *Lily of the valley is a powerful herb and must only be prescribed by a professional herbalist.*

Taking herbal remedies

ABOVE: **Herbal tinctures and lozenges.** *Tinctures are made by steeping herbs in alcohol.*

THE LEAF, ROOT, STEM, *flower, seed, fruit, or bark of a plant may be included in a herbal preparation. The prescription may be given in a variety of forms, including the fresh herb, loose dried plant parts, tea, tincture, decoction, cream, syrup, wash, capsules, tablets, pills, gargle, poultice, suppositories, inhalant, pessaries, rub, douche, fomentation, and compress.*

ABOVE: **Herbal tablets and capsules.** *You can buy empty capsules from pharmacists, to fill with your own herbal remedy.*

Some prescriptions may involve taking a simple herb-filled capsule 3 times a day, while others may require the herb to be boiled for 20 minutes and then drunk 4 times daily. Some herbalists may even grow, pick, and prepare their own remedies. The method depends on the condition to be treated, the

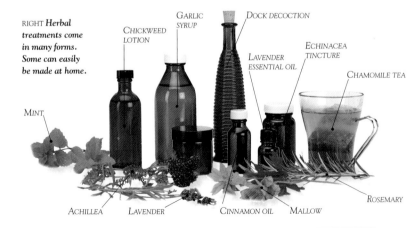

RIGHT **Herbal treatments come in many forms. Some can easily be made at home.**

GARLIC SYRUP

CHICKWEED LOTION

DOCK DECOCTION

LAVENDER ESSENTIAL OIL

ECHINACEA TINCTURE

CHAMOMILE TEA

MINT

ACHILLEA

LAVENDER

CINNAMON OIL

MALLOW

ROSEMARY

approach of the herbalist and the situation of the patient, and their level of commitment and interest. Sometimes there is a choice of methods. Most herbalists will be happy to explain what is in their medicine.

HOW TO TAKE YOUR MEDICINE

☞ Herbs, like all medicines, should be taken regularly and the course completed as prescribed.

☞ Never share prescribed medicines. A remedy from a professional herbalist is a unique and personal medicine, specifically for you and your situation. It may not be suitable for another person. Recommend the herbalist, not the medicine.

LENGTH OF TREATMENT

The length of treatment depends on the ailment. Acute conditions should respond in a few days, chronic long-term conditions may need treatment lasting several months before a pronounced improvement is felt.

Do regular maintenance tests to monitor improvement. It is a good idea to check the body

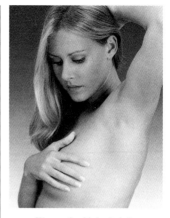

ABOVE: *Women should check their breasts regularly. It is also a good idea to periodically check other parts of the body.*

yearly to make sure that muscle tone, joint mobility, lung capacity, and recovery rate are maintained at your optimum. This personal self-examination routine can easily be added to breast and scrotum checks.

HERBAL PREPARATIONS

☞ 1 cup of herb tea 3–6 times a day – the standard treatment.

☞ 1 teaspoon of tincture (the herb preserved in alcohol) 3 times a day.

☞ Drops, plant juices, fluid extract, and glycerine extracts are popular, as are capsules and compressed tablets.

MATERIA
MEDICA

Yarrow

ACHILLEA MILLEFOLIUM

The following pages list 25 of the most useful, common herbs for home treatment. They are freely available: some are common wild plants, others can be grown in gardens or window boxes, but most can be obtained from shops. They are simple to use and effective if dispensed sensibly and as directed.

A COMMON WEED *found growing in grassy places and lawns, with feathery leaves and small pink or white flowers. The whole plant is picked in full flower.*

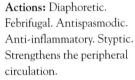

Actions: Diaphoretic. Febrifugal. Antispasmodic. Anti-inflammatory. Styptic. Strengthens the peripheral circulation.

Indications: Fevers, colds, and flu. Can be used for children's fever, diarrhea, and stomach cramps. Stops bleeding and promotes healing of wounds. Erratic and heavy periods.

Contraindications: Avoid large doses in pregnancy.

Method and dose: The tea may be taken freely in acute conditions. To strengthen circulation take 3 cups a day.

COMMENTS

The fresh root is a good analgesic for toothache. The herbal tea is specific for the early stages of fevers.

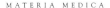

Mallow

ALTHAEA OFFICINALIS

ABOVE: *Mallow leaves should be collected after the plant has flowered in summer.*

A BEAUTIFUL WILD PLANT *with pale pink flowers.* Althaea officinalis *is the marsh mallow. Other species may be used. Despite its name, marsh mallow may be grown in gardens.*

Actions: Demulcent, soothing and healing.

Indications: Soothes and heals ulcers, inflammations of the digestive tract, dry and unproductive coughs, cystitis, and bladder irritations. Draws abscesses, bites, and stings. Dries and soothes wet eczema.

Contraindications: None.

Method and dose: The leaf may be taken freely as a tea. It is often mixed with other herbs, for example with thyme for unproductive coughs, and with bearberry for cystitis. Mix the powdered root of mallow into a thick paste with a little water to draw bites, stings, and splinters.

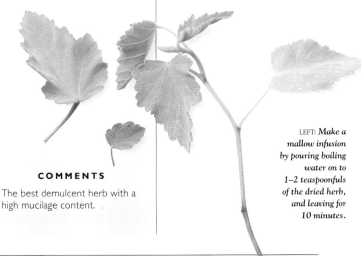

LEFT: *Make a mallow infusion by pouring boiling water on to 1–2 teaspoonfuls of the dried herb, and leaving for 10 minutes.*

COMMENTS

The best demulcent herb with a high mucilage content.

Celery seed

APIUM GRAVEOLENS

THE SEEDS *of the common garden vegetable. Collect them when ripe in the fall.*

ABOVE: *Celery juice can be drunk before a meal to suppress the appetite.*

Actions: Diuretic, urinary antiseptic, carminative, digestive, antiseptic, and anti-depressive.

Indications: Rheumatism, arthritis; and gout. Cystitis and flatulence. Aids milk flow in nursing mothers. As a mouthwash for bad breath.

Contraindications: Avoid in pregnancy.

Method and dose: For a decoction: use ½ teaspoon of crushed seeds to 1 cup of water. Tincture: use ½ teaspoonful (2ml), taken 3 times daily. Combines well with willow bark for arthritic conditions.

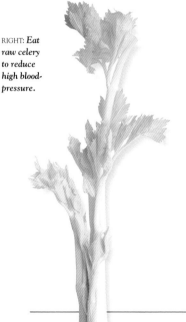

RIGHT: *Eat raw celery to reduce high blood-pressure.*

COMMENTS

Specific for arthritis with depression. Celery itself has similar properties and may be eaten, or the juice taken, to back up the actions of the seeds. Do not use seeds bought for planting.

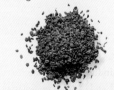

ABOVE: **Celery seeds are rich in iron and vitamins A, B, and C.**

Marigold

CALENDULA OFFICINALIS

THE POT MARIGOLD. *A popular garden plant with bright orange or yellow flowers. Easily grown and self-seeds readily.*

RIGHT: **Calendula is especially good for treating a child with a fever and swollen neck glands.**

Actions: Lymphatic deobstructant, alterative, anti-inflammatory, antiseptic, and anti-fungal. Antispasmodic.

Indications: Swollen lymph glands, mumps, pelvic congestion, infections, and inflammations in general. Prevents period pains. Skin diseases, wounds, cuts, stings, and swellings. Varicose veins, chapped skin, and thrush.

Contraindications: None.

Method and dose: The tea may be taken freely. Lotions, creams, and compresses for wounds and inflammations of the skin. Compresses for the eyes. Infused oil for dry skin and chapped lips. Also gargles, mouthwashes, and baths.

COMMENTS

Often sold as calendula. Do not confuse with French and African marigolds (*Tagetes*), which should not be taken internally.

RIGHT: **Marigold petals should be dried carefully after picking.**

Cayenne

CAPSICUM MINIMUM

THE COMMON RED HOT *chilli pepper, used as a kitchen spice. There are many different types.*

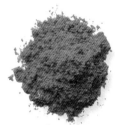

ABOVE: *Cayenne pepper can be used to make an infused oil to warm the joints and soothe muscle spasm.*

Actions: Warming, stimulant, circulatory stimulant, carminative. Useful topical analgesic.

Indications: Poor circulation, low energy, failing digestion in old people. Impotence. As a cream or oil for unbroken chilblains, lower back pain, and post-shingles neuralgia.

Contraindications: Large doses may irritate the stomach in susceptible people.

Method and dose: Best used as a tincture. Add 1 or 2 drops to herbal teas or tinctures, every few hours if necessary. Use the cream on small areas only.

LEFT: *As in cooking, use cayenne in very small quantities.*

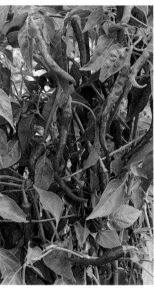

ABOVE: *Cayenne can be used as a general tonic, but works especially well on the circulatory and digestive systems.*

COMMENTS

Especially useful for elderly people and those who feel the cold easily.

Cinnamon

CINNAMOMUM ZEYLANICUM

THE AROMATIC BARK *of a tree commonly grown in Sri Lanka. A common spice in the kitchen.*

Actions: Warming, antispasmodic, antiseptic, carminative. Promotes digestion and lifts the spirits.

Indications: Weak digestion, poor appetite, acidity, colds, and fevers. Helps general debility and weakness.

Contraindications: None.

Method and dose: Add an inch (2cm) of cinnamon quill, or a good pinch of the powder, to teas for colds and fevers. Chew a piece of quill for head colds. Add 10–20 drops of the tincture to any medicine for poor digestion or debility. Makes a good massage oil for weak chests.

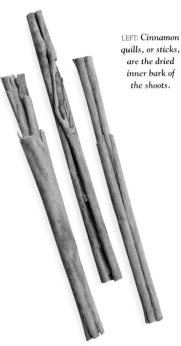

LEFT: *Cinnamon quills, or sticks, are the dried inner bark of the shoots.*

GROUND CINNAMON

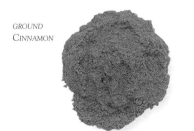

COMMENTS

The whole quills are better than the powder. Specific for coldness and weakness. Much more gentle to use than cayenne.

Hawthorn

CRATAEGUS MONOGYNA,
CRATAEGUS OXYACANTHOIDES

HAWTHORN IS THE *"May blossom tree,"* commonly seen in hedgerows. It is also often grown in parks and gardens. The berries or the flowering tops are used.

Actions: Heart restorative, lowers blood-pressure, and clears blood vessels. Antispasmodic.

Indications: Strengthens failing hearts in old people and in those recovering from disease. Moderately raised blood-pressure, arteriosclerosis, white finger, insomnia, and colic.

Contraindications: Potentiates dioxin. Heart disease should be treated by a professional.

Method and dose: Berries as a decoction or tops as a tea, 3 cups daily. Tincture: 3–4 teaspoons daily. Continue to take for at least 6 months.

COMMENTS

Specific for strengthening the heart. Complements most other medicines but suspected heart problems should always be checked out by a professional.

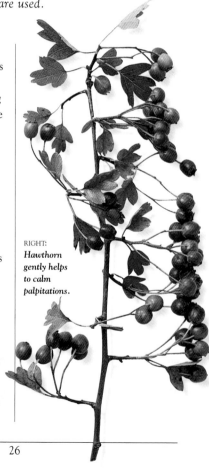

RIGHT:
Hawthorn gently helps to calm palpitations.

Echinacea

ECHINACEA ANGUSTIFOLIA,
ECHINACEA PURPUREA

A LARGE-FLOWERED *purple daisy. A native of the US some-times known as the purple cone flower. Both flower and root may be used.*

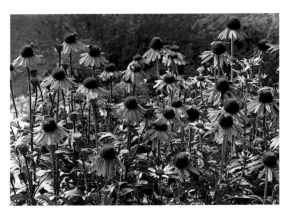

LEFT: *Echinacea roots should be dug up in the fall, and are best used fresh for decoctions.*

Actions: Alterative, blood cleanser, antiseptic. Stimulates the immune system.
Indications: Boils, abscesses, infected spots, duodenal ulcers, herpes, influenza, and infections in general. Infected sore throats and gum disease.
Contraindications: None.
Method and dose: ½ cup of decoction or 1 teaspoon of tincture 4–5 times daily for 2 weeks, when needed. Mix 1 teaspoon of tincture in ½ cup of water for a gargle.

COMMENTS

Echinacea is best taken in high doses for short periods. Tablets and capsules are widely available. Goes well with garlic.

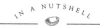
St. John's wort

HYPERICUM PERFORATUM

A WILD PLANT *commonly found on alkaline soils. It grows to about 15in (60cm) and has pretty yellow flowers. The top part of the plant is picked in full flower. There are several different species, so make sure you pick the correct one.*

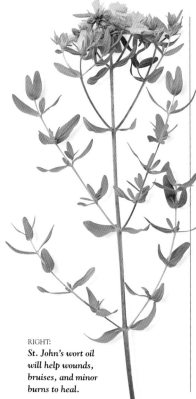

RIGHT:
St. John's wort oil will help wounds, bruises, and minor burns to heal.

Actions: Nervine. Antidepressant and antiinflammatory.

Indications: Mild depression and anxiety. Neurasthenia and organic nerve diseases. Neuralgia, nerve pains, and back pains. Puncture wounds.

Contraindications: Don't treat severe depression.

Method and dose: 2–3 cups of tea or 3–4 teaspoons of the tincture daily. The sun-infused oil is an excellent massage for nerve pain and makes a good base carrier for essential oils.

COMMENTS

Concentrated extracts are now available on the market: taken in large doses, these may cause a rash after exposure to sunshine.

Juniper

JUNIPERUS COMMUNIS

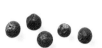

ABOVE: *Pick plump, ripe juniper berries in the fall, and dry them slowly.*

THE AROMATIC BERRIES *of a small evergreen tree, often grown in gardens or ornamental parks. The berries are rich in essential oil, are also used in cooking, and for making gin.*

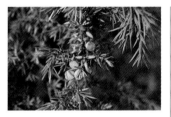

ABOVE: *Juniper is a hardy evergreen, tolerant of a variety of conditions. The leaves are aromatic when crushed.*

Actions: Stimulant diuretic. Urinary antiseptic. A good digestive tonic.

Indications: Cystitis with catarrh, arthritis, and rheumatism. Locally for slow-to-heal wounds, aches, and pains.

Contraindications: Avoid in pregnancy, and when suffering from kidney disease.

Method and dose: Make the tea with ½ teaspoon of crushed berries to a cup of boiling water. Infuse for 15 minutes. Take 2–3 cups a day. This strength of tea can be used as a wash for slow-to-heal wounds and as a hand bath for stiff and painful joints. Also used as a massage oil.

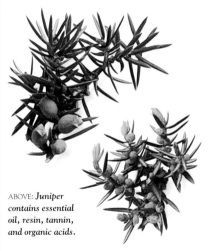

ABOVE: *Juniper contains essential oil, resin, tannin, and organic acids.*

COMMENTS

Specific for arthritic aches and pains.

Chamomile

MATRICARIA RECUTITA

A SMALL WILD DAISY WITH FEATHERY LEAVES *and distinctive smell. The flowers are used. Both German chamomile* (Matricaria recutita) *and garden chamomile* (Chamaemelum nobile) *are suitable.*

Actions: Anti-inflammatory, antispasmodic, carminative, mild sedative. Very soothing for any irritating conditions.

Indications: Digestive disorders. Headaches, stress, irritability, nervousness, and allergies of all kinds. Itchy and inflamed skin conditions.

Contraindications: None.

Method and dose: Chamomile is a very versatile herb. The tea may be taken freely. As a cream, lotion, or compress. Cold, spent tea bags can be used for cooling sore eyes.

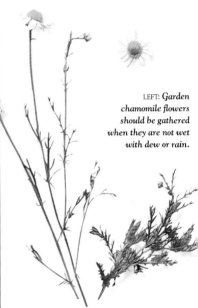

LEFT: *Garden chamomile flowers should be gathered when they are not wet with dew or rain.*

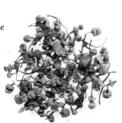

RIGHT: *Dried chamomile can be combined with linden and clove to make a delicious tea to help promote restful sleep.*

COMMENTS

Although chamomile comes in tea bags, it is best to prepare it in a closed vessel to retain the aromatic oils. Chamomile tea is suitable for restless children and teething troubles.

Lemon balm

MELISSA OFFICINALIS

A VIGOROUS GARDEN *perennial that is easily grown. Bees love it. The stalks, leaves, and flowers are used and picked as it comes into flower.*

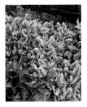

ABOVE: **Melissa** *is derived from the Greek word for "bee."*

Actions: Antispasmodic and anti-depressant. Carminative and relaxing. Locally antiviral.

Indications: Nervous indigestion, depression, and low spirits, insomnia, nightmares, and general excitability. The cold tea is cooling in hot weather.

Contraindications: None.

Method and dose: To get the full aromatic properties of the plant, it is best to take the fresh plant as a tea. Fresh plant tinctures are also useful.

COMMENTS

The tea taken every morning with a little honey added is strengthening in convalescence and for the elderly.

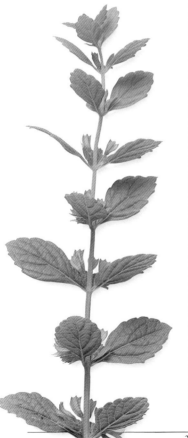

LEFT: *Sprigs of lemon balm are traditionally placed in beehives to calm restless bees.*

Parsley

PETROSELINUM CRISPUM

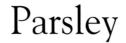

PARSLEY IS A COMMON *garden herb. The leaf is used. The curled-leaf variety is best for herbalism.*

ABOVE: **Parsley flowers. Parsley attracts bees and may repel aphids.**

Actions: Diuretic, tonic, nourishing, and carminative.

Indications: Painful urination and water retention, especially when premenstrual. Women's tonic for menstrual problems and at the menopause. Fatigue and general weakness. Depression. Gas and digestive weakness.

Contraindications: Avoid in pregnancy and kidney disease. Parsley seed is toxic and should not be taken internally.

Method and dose: The tea may be taken 3–4 times daily. Add chopped fresh parsley to salads. It is rich in minerals, including calcium and iron.

COMMENTS

An excellent tonic for older menopausal women.

ABOVE: *Fresh parsley will contribute a rich source of vitamin C if you include it in your diet.*

Raspberry

RUBUS IDAEUS

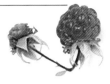

A POPULAR SOFT FRUIT, *easily grown, and also found in the wild. The leaves and fruit are used.*

ABOVE: *Different varieties of raspberry bear fruit in the summer or the fall.*

Actions: Astringent tonic for the womb, mouth, and bowels.
Indications: Diarrhea, and nervous diarrhea with mucus. Sores and thrush in the mouth. Pregnancy.
Contraindications: None.
Method and dose: Raspberries soaked in cider vinegar are used as a gargle, a cooling summer drink, and as a good source of vitamin C – particularly in the winter months. Take 1–2 dessert-spoonfuls in a glass of water, depending on taste. The leaves are taken as a tea, 3 cups a day.

COMMENTS

Three cups of tea a day taken during the last 3 months of pregnancy will strengthen the womb and help at the birth. Continue taking after the birth to restore womb tone quickly.

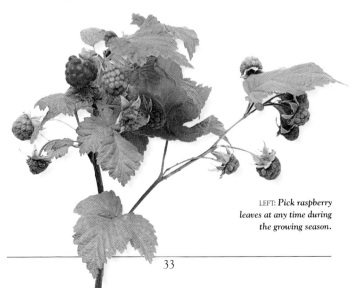

LEFT: *Pick raspberry leaves at any time during the growing season.*

Dock

RUMEX CRISPUS

ABOVE: **Dried yellow dock root. Clean and split the root before drying.**

A LARGE-LEAFED, *common weed of wayside and wasteland. The root is generally used. Rumex crispus is yellow dock. Other species may be used.*

Actions: Alterative, laxative, and generally cooling.

Indications: Mild jaundice, "liverishness," chronic skin conditions, chronic constipation, rheumatism, and skin infections (topically). The leaves of dock are used to take the heat out of nettle stings.

Contraindications: None.

Method and dose: Make a decoction with ½oz (12.5g) root to 1 pint (500ml) of water. Take ½ cup, 3 times daily.

COMMENTS

Many chronic skin conditions respond to a combination of dock and burdock roots. Take 3 cups of the decoction daily for some months.

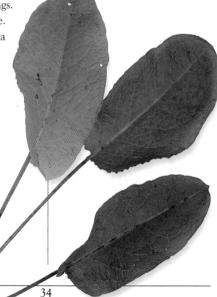

RIGHT: **The broad-leaved dock,** Rumex obtusifolius, **is also suitable for herbal use.**

Sage

SALVIA OFFICINALIS

SAGE IS A SMALL BUSH *from southern Europe, and a common garden plant. It is often regarded as mainly a culinary herb. The leaves are used. The volatile oils in sage will soothe the mucous membranes of the mouth and throat.*

Actions: Tonic, antiseptic, antispasmodic, carminative. Said to promote long life. Reduces breast milk.

Indications: Sore throat, laryngitis, mouth, and gum disease. Night sweats. Loss of appetite and indigestion. Painful swollen breasts. Depression and hot flushes during menopause. Poor memory. Helpful in diabetes. Restorative following viral infections.

Contraindications: Pregnancy and nursing.

Method and dose: The tea may be taken 3 times daily for long-term use. Use cold tea for hot flushes and night sweats. Make a strong tea with a little honey for gargles and mouthwashes. Creams for eczema.

LEFT: *Make a sage compress to help with the healing of wounds.*

COMMENTS

Specific for the menopause. A useful pick-me-up.

Elderflower

SAMBUCUS NIGRA

A SMALL TREE *with pretty white flowers carried in flat masses. Common in woods, hedgerows, and wasteland. The flowers, bark, berries, and leaves have useful properties.*

Actions: Diaphoretic, gentle diuretic, restores and tones mucous membranes.

Indications: The common cold, influenza, and fevers in general. Nasal catarrh, sinusitis, rhinitis, and hay fever.

Contraindications: None.

Method and dose: The tea may be drunk freely for colds and fevers. Take 3 cups of tea daily for preventing recurrent colds and hay fever – start 2 months before the pollen season. Well-strained tea can be used as a wash for sore and inflamed eyes.

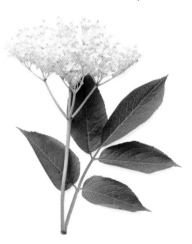

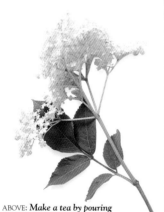

ABOVE: *Make a tea by pouring boiling water onto 2 teaspoonfuls of fresh or dried elderflowers.*

COMMENTS

Specific for colds with a dripping nose. Makes a useful tea for children's fevers.

Chickweed

STELLARIA MEDIA

A LOW-GROWING, *soft plant that grows as a common weed. The whole plant is used externally to treat cuts, and to relieve the itching caused by eczema and psoriasis.*

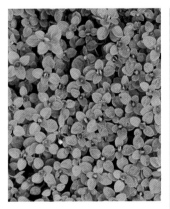

ABOVE: *A strong infusion of chickweed can be added to a bath to soothe itchy skin.*

COMMENTS

When it is green and fresh, add it to "spring-cleaning" tea, or drink freely to cool when feverish. The fresh leaves, as a poultice, will gently draw spots and small boils. As a cream or wash it is useful for piles, hot and irritating itches, and sunburn. Nourishing in salads because of its mineral content.

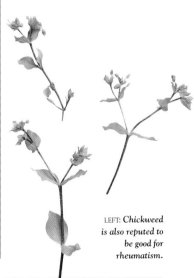

Actions: Cooling, demulcent, and relieves itching. Mild alterative.

Indications: Boils, varicose ulcers, inflamed joints, eczema, and contact dermatitis.

Contraindications: None.

Method and dose: Works particularly well as a lotion, ointment, and compress.

LEFT: *Chickweed is also reputed to be good for rheumatism.*

Comfrey

SYMPHYTUM OFFICINALE

A LARGE, hairy wild plant, commonly found in damp soil. It has beautiful purple bell-shaped flowers. The flowering tops are used.

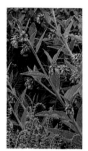

ABOVE:
Make comfrey ointment by adding beeswax to comfrey leaf-infused oil.

Actions:
Demulcent and promotes healing, internally and externally.

Indications:
Wounds, cuts, and sprains. Broken bones and arthritis. Stomach ulcers and inflammations of the digestive tract. Persistent coughs.

Contraindications: Best avoided in pregnancy and infancy.

Method and dose:
Local use as a cream or a compress, and in liniments. Drink 1 cup of tea 3 times a day. Use in syrups for dry coughs.

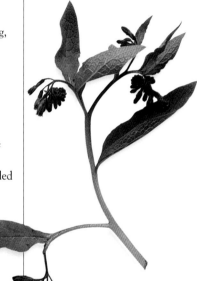

RIGHT: *Comfrey is a very good plant to use as a green manure: the plant is dug back into the soil to improve fertility.*

COMMENTS

There has been some controversy over comfrey, and the internal use of the root has been discontinued except in professional practice. Teas made from the green parts are safe.

Dandelion

TARAXACUM OFFICINALIS

THE COMMON WEED *of lawns and wayside. Most gardeners spend a lot of time trying to eradicate its deep tap roots! Leaves, roots, and flowers are used.*

ABOVE: **Dried dandelion root. Collect roots between early and late summer.**

Actions: The root is mildly laxative and strengthens the liver. The leaves are diuretic.

Indications: The root for mild jaundice, gallstones, general "liverishness," poor appetite, allergies and food sensitivities, skin complaints, and rheumatism. The leaf for water retention, swollen ankles, premenstrual water retention, and with urinary antiseptics for cystitis. The sap from the flower stalk can be applied to warts.

Contraindications: Avoid diuretic teas if taking "water tablets" on prescription.

Method and dose: May be taken freely. The root is decocted and the leaf taken as a tea. Dandelion "coffee" is made by roasting the root, and makes a passable substitute for coffee. The fresh leaves are a delicious addition to salads.

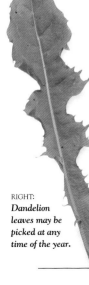

RIGHT:
Dandelion leaves may be picked at any time of the year.

COMMENTS

Suitable for any condition that requires cleansing of the system. The common dandelion is a treasure, don't decry it as merely a weed.

Thyme

THYMUS VULGARIS

THYME IS A *low-growing garden herb. Many varieties are grown and most may be used medicinally. Pick the short stalks just before flowering.*

BELOW: *Thyme tea can help to alleviate an asthma attack.*

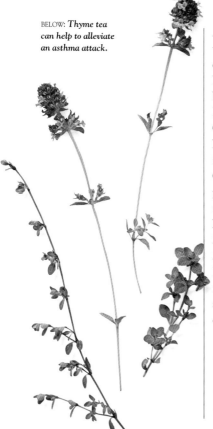

Actions: Antiseptic, anti-fungal, vermifugal, stimulant expectorant, relaxes the bronchi.
Indications: Lung infections, bronchitis, and whooping cough. Irritable bowel. Intestinal worms. Cystitis and bedwetting. Nightmares. Cuts and fungal infections.
Contraindications: Avoid in pregnancy. The amounts taken in food are safe.
Method and dose: 3 cups of tea, 3–4 dessertspoonfuls of syrup, or 3–4 teaspoons of tincture daily. Double the dose for acute chest infections. Excellent chest rub and inhalant. Bath, lotion, and cream for fungal infections.

COMMENTS

An excellent antiseptic. Specific for lung infections.

Lime flower

TILIA EUROPAEA

A HANDSOME TREE *often planted in streets and parks. The flowers are used, picked with their bracts in June, just as their flowering period ends.*

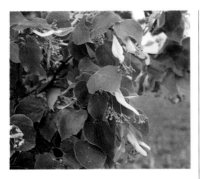

ABOVE: *Lime flower's relaxing effects aid the treatment of certain types of migraine.*

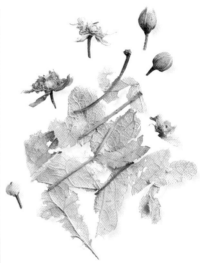

ABOVE: *An infusion from dried lime flowers may be added to a baby's bath to improve eczema.*

Actions: Sedative nerve tonic.
Anti-spasmodic.
Diaphoretic.

Indications:
Anxiety, insomnia, and restless excitability. A helpful adjunct in high blood-pressure and the early stages of flu and fevers.

Contraindications: None.

Method and dose: Drink the tea 3 times a day. It makes a pleasant everyday drink and it is a good herb to start with for those unfamiliar with herb teas.

COMMENTS

Lime combines well with other herbs: lime and balm for coping with stress, lime and peppermint for the relief of digestive disorders.

Nettle

URTICA DIOICA

THE UBIQUITOUS *stinging nettle. The young leaves are best.*

Actions: Tonic, iron tonic, restores and cleanses the blood, mild diuretic.

Indications: Iron-deficiency anemia, exhaustion, and lethargy. Excellent for pregnancy and nursing, ensuring adequate iron levels, and good milk supply. Hair loss. Nettle rash and nervous eczema. The roots are helpful for treating the swelling of the prostate.

Contraindications: None.

Method and dose: The tea may be taken freely. For anemia, use in soups or cook as spinach and eat daily to ensure a high enough dosage.
Make a strong tea or a vinegar extract to use as a hair rinse.

COMMENTS

Specific for lethargy in springtime. To ensure a constant crop of young leaves, keep cutting the patch back.

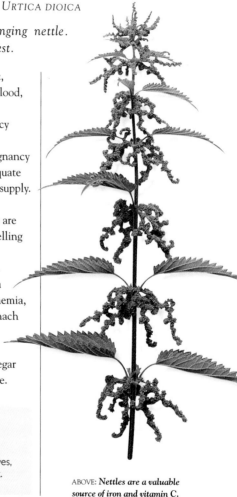

ABOVE: **Nettles are a valuable source of iron and vitamin C.**

Ginger

ZINGIBER OFFICINALE

A TROPICAL PLANT. *The root is used as a popular kitchen spice.*

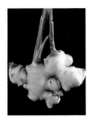

ABOVE: *The rhizome, or enlarged underground stem, of the ginger plant is used.*

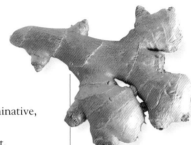

LEFT: *A gargle with ginger decoction may improve a sore throat.*

Actions: Warming, antispasmodic, carminative, anti-emetic. Gentle circulatory stimulant.

Indications: Nausea, travel sickness, the nausea of pregnancy, loss of appetite, poor digestion, and hiccups. Chills and feelings of cold. Period pains.

Contraindications: None.

Method and dose: 10 drops of tincture in any herb tea or mixed with a little honey on a spoon. Grated root made into a tea may be drunk freely for pains and chills. Candied ginger and powdered ginger in capsules are handy preparations for nausea.

COMMENTS

Specific for chills and for nausea from any cause. Thinly sliced fresh root is better than the powder for most uses.

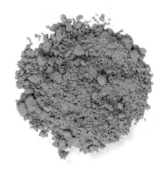

RIGHT: *Powdered ginger. The warming qualities of ginger oil are beneficial in massage.*

Herbal medicine in the home

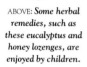

THIS BOOK CONCENTRATES ON *herbs which are freely available over the counter or growing wild. Many recipes are traditional and have been used successfully generation after generation. They are still in use because they work.*

ABOVE: *Some herbal remedies, such as these eucalyptus and honey lozenges, are enjoyed by children.*

The aim of home treatment is to help support the body, speed recovery, and make the condition as comfortable as possible. Herbs are especially useful for children to help them through the minor infections of childhood, and to ensure a strong constitution. Herbal medicine is also an excellent support for the elderly and convalescents.

RIGHT: *A vaporizer heats oil to release herbal vapors into the air.*

THE PRINCIPLES OF HOME TREATMENT

- Act immediately.
- Know why you are taking a herb and what to expect.
- Choose the most suitable method: tea, tincture, bath, etc.
- Monitor the response.
- Don't be impatient. Be prepared to continue treatment over several months for long-term conditions.
- Use plenty of tender loving care. This is an important aspect of home care.
- If the condition worsens or suddenly changes, seek professional assistance.
- Keep notes so that your skill and expertise grow. This will also be useful if you need to seek outside assistance.
- Do not panic at any diagnosis. Herbal remedies can contribute toward well-being in any situation. They can even be helpful for terminal conditions.

For example, a terminally ill patient can be soothed in the following ways:

☞ Soak or gently massage the hands or feet with infused oil of lavender or chamomile.

☞ Wipe the brow with a cloth dipped in chamomile, lavender, or linden tea.

☞ In dry, centrally heated rooms, spray the air with peppermint, rosemary, or lavender tea to ease the patient's breathing.

THE ELDERLY

Herbal tonics are ideal for the elderly, and it is a good idea to drink a tonic tea each day at breakfast time. Herbs such as lemon balm, chamomile, peppermint, sage, rosemary, and basil all have useful benefits to offer when used singly or in combination.

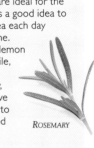

ROSEMARY

PREGNANCY

There are many herbs which are safe to use during pregnancy but it is best to seek professional guidance for any condition which needs new treatment. Personal health regimes, such as chamomile and linden tea daily, can be maintained.

☞ Raspberry strengthens the womb if taken in the last trimester.

☞ Clove tea can be taken immediately contractions start and throughout labor for pain.

☞ Ginseng can be chewed for energy if labor is protracted and exhausting.

☞ Nursing mothers should also seek advice before responding to a new condition or changing their herbal routine.

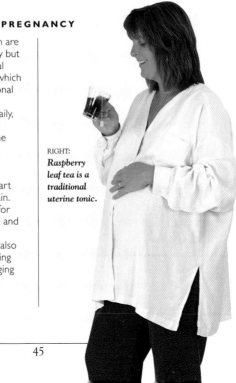

RIGHT:
Raspberry leaf tea is a traditional uterine tonic.

A HOME HERBAL MEDICINE CHEST

Herbs lose their freshness so they must be replaced each season. For convenience some herbs may need to be turned into syrups or infused oils.

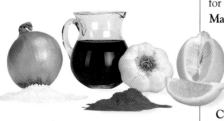

ABOVE: *You will already have some ingredients on your kitchen shelves.*

☞ Remember the healing ingredients already in the kitchen: salt, pepper, lemon, onions, garlic, and vinegar. From these it is possible to start immediate treatment. Weak salt water is unbeatable as an eyewash and as a cleansing wash for abrasions and wounds. A pinch of cayenne pepper can be added to a cup of tea to ward off chills and warm a chilled body.

☞ Buy a simple first-aid box with scissors, tweezers, eyebath, and an assortment of bandages and plasters, to be ready for all occasions.

COLLECT THE FOLLOWING

Rescue Remedy: This is a Bach Flower Remedy. Also available as Five Flower Remedy. Take immediately for all forms of shock, accident, or trauma. Safe for children and animals.

Marigold tincture. For cuts and spots. As a cool compress for heat, sprains, and swellings. As a gargle for a sore throat. For mild fevers: 1 teaspoon 3 times a day.

Cold and flu tea: Elderflower, peppermint, and yarrow. Drink a cup 3–4 times a day.

Ginger tincture: A few drops in hot water, or any tea, will calm nausea, relax spasms, and warm you up. Add 1 drop to 1fl oz (25ml) oil and ¾ fl oz (20ml) water to make a liniment for cold, cramped muscles and menstrual spasms.

Clove oil: For toothache, add 3 drops to water for an antiseptic mouthwash, gargle, or wash for wounds. For muscular aches, add 10 drops to 1fl oz (25ml) of sunflower oil and massage in well.

GINGER

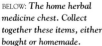
BELOW: *The home herbal medicine chest. Collect together these items, either bought or homemade.*

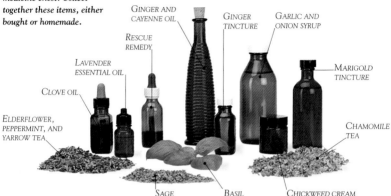

GINGER AND CAYENNE OIL

RESCUE REMEDY

GINGER TINCTURE

GARLIC AND ONION SYRUP

LAVENDER ESSENTIAL OIL

MARIGOLD TINCTURE

CLOVE OIL

ELDERFLOWER, PEPPERMINT, AND YARROW TEA

CHAMOMILE TEA

SAGE

BASIL

CHICKWEED CREAM

"Hot" oil: An infused oil of ginger and cayenne is an excellent standby for cramps, spasm, and muscular aches. Rub in well and then take a salt bath. Also for chilblains and poor circulation to the feet.

Chickweed or marigold cream: For dry, chapped, irritated skin and piles.

Restorative tea: Use two-thirds sage to one-third basil.

Calming tea: Chamomile tea for restlessness. Chamomile, linden, and clove for restful sleep.

Lavender essential oil: Diluted in water as an antiseptic wash for all wounds. As a cool compress for headaches and tired eyes. For stress, 2 drops in warm water is a calming restorative. Put 3 drops on a pillow to bring restful sleep.

Sage: As a gargle and mouthwash for sore throats. As a hot tea for fevers.

Chamomile: This has many uses, but above all it is a digestive.

Cough remedy: The best are garlic and onion syrups, or alternatively chamomile and thyme.

LAVENDER

SAGE

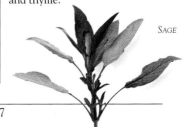

Common ailments

BELOW ARE LISTED *some of the common health problems that can be treated at home with herbal remedies.*

COLDS

☞ The traditional "cold and flu" tea is exceptionally effective when taken promptly, as it treats all elements of a cold. Use equal amounts of elderflower, peppermint, and yarrow, brewed as a tea and taken freely, from 3–6 cups a day.

☞ If the body is chilled, add a pinch of a warming remedy such as ginger.

☞ If there is restlessness, add chamomile.

COUGHS

☞ Coughs can be wet and productive or dry and irritating, depending on the cause.

☞ Stimulating expectorants such as thyme and garlic clear stubborn phlegm and fight infection.

☞ Add soothing herbs such as licorice, coltsfoot, and comfrey for raw and irritating coughs.

☞ Use chest rubs made with essential or infused oils of thyme, eucalyptus, or garlic.

THYME

ASTHMA

☞ Chronic conditions like asthma respond best to professional treatment. Home aids include keeping the air damp, and soothing the airways with an inhalant of essential oils in steam or an oil burner.

☞ Lavender is calming, thyme and aniseed clear phlegm and relax the airways.

☞ Thyme tea with honey is also very helpful for asthmatics.

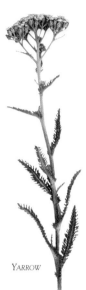

FEVERS

☞ The body raises its temperature in an effort to eliminate the infection.

☞ Diaphoretic herbs which induce sweating, such as sage, catmint, elderflower, and yarrow, should be taken freely as hot teas.

☞ Use cooling compresses or washes, such as cider vinegar in water, to bring down high temperatures.

YARROW

HEADACHES

☞ Stress headaches can be relieved by drinking strong chamomile tea.

☞ Rosemary tea is best for headaches linked with stomach troubles. Feverfew products are specific for migraine.

☞ Compresses on the forehead or at the back of the neck can often be useful.

☞ Use lavender or neroli oils diluted in water.

FLU

☞ Treat as for colds, see above.

☞ Influenza is caused by a virus. It should be treated seriously or it will hang on and cause debility and depression.

☞ Do not work through it, allow time to recover.

☞ Take echinacea products to boost the immune system and drink sage tea for recovery.

HAY FEVER

☞ Strengthen resistance with a tea of elderflowers and yarrow for some weeks before the pollen season starts.

☞ Soothe itchy eyes with an elderflower, eyebright, or chamomile compress. Eyebright tea or capsules will relieve symptoms.

☞ A teaspoon of local honey, before and during the season, helps many people.

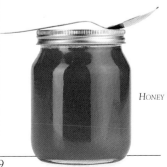

HONEY

HAIR LOSS AND BALDNESS

👁 Hereditary male baldness is intractable, but much can be done to improve the quality of the scalp and reduce premature hair loss.

👁 Improve circulation to the head by drinking rosemary tea every day. Massage the scalp with infused ginger or fenugreek oils. Then rinse with nettle vinegar.

GINGER

DANDRUFF

👁 Improve circulation to the scalp. Rosemary is the herb of choice taken internally as a tea and used as an application. For dry hair, rub rosemary-infused oil into the scalp before washing. For greasy hair, add rosemary vinegar or a few drops of rosemary essential oil to the rinsing water.

ECZEMA

👁 Strong marigold or chamomile tea, used as a lotion or added to the bath for infants, is soothing.

👁 Avoid soap. Instead, use emollient creams for washing. For dry skin, apply marigold-infused oil after bathing.

👁 A useful herb tea mixture can be made from equal parts of dandelion root, burdock root, and red clover flowers.

COLD SORES

👁 Act immediately the first tingle is felt.

👁 St. John's wort tincture, applied immediately, should prevent the incipient cold sore from coming to fruition.

👁 Once the sore is established, myrrh tincture can be applied sparingly to dry it up. Check general health and reduce overall stress levels.

👁 Cold sores are infectious – wash hands carefully after applying any lotion, and only use a personal towel.

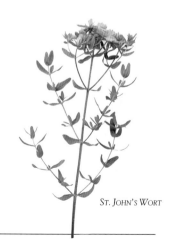

ST. JOHN'S WORT

ALLERGIES

☞ Avoid known allergens.

☞ Strengthen the weakened area with tonic teas, 2 cups taken over a period of time (the sinuses with elderflower tea, the stomach with chamomile, linden, and a warming digestive like cardamom, the skin with chamomile washes and rosemary in the bath).

☞ If suffering a sudden allergic reaction, take Rescue Remedy (*see* p. 46).

CELLULITE

☞ Cellulite will respond to massage, skin brushing, and plenty of fluids.

☞ Massage with juniper-infused oil and take a cleansing tea of herbs such as marigold.

DEPRESSION

☞ A good tea to balance mind and body is lemon balm.

☞ Look to the causes of the depression, and your general health.

☞ Mild depression is a natural response to many difficult life events such as birth and death.

☞ Seek help if the condition persists.

FAINTING

☞ Loosen clothing around the neck and revive with a whiff of rosemary essential oil, or the fresh herb crushed.

☞ Then get the patient to drink a cup of chamomile tea with a small pinch of cayenne.

In older people fainting may be associated with heart or circulatory problems, which should be investigated.

NEURALGIA

☞ Ask a dentist to check your teeth, bite, and jaw alignment.

☞ Make a massage oil with rosemary and lavender essential oils. These herbs can also be drunk as teas.

☞ Chamomile is effective.

A compress of warm cider vinegar can bring relief.

☞ Rub in cayenne-infused oil for cold and post-shingles neuralgia.

LEFT: *Massage using essential oils benefits many conditions, including neuralgia, rheumatism, and arthritis.*

INSOMNIA

☞ Chamomile tea is best for mild restlessness, as it warms the stomach and the body, and therefore relaxes you.

☞ A tea made with equal parts of chamomile and linden flowers is effective. Add 4 cloves for their analgesic effect if needed.

☞ Use lavender or hop pillows.

☞ Insomnia is quite common during periods of stress. Try not to worry about it.

Lavender

STRESS

☞ Lots of things in life cause stress, aggravation, and tension. The trick is to learn how to manage it and not let it build up.

☞ Relaxing teas such as chamomile and linden, lavender baths, meditation, regular exercise, yoga, and allowing space for yourself are all useful techniques for managing stress.

CHRONIC FATIGUE SYNDROME, OR ME

☞ ME, like most chronic conditions, should be treated professionally. Home aids include sage and echinacea to maintain strength, St. John's wort or cardamom to lift depression, and cinnamon for warming.

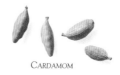

Cardamom

☞ Pace yourself, set realistic goals, and guard against depression. Lavender or thyme oils in the bath ease aching muscles.

☞ Deep breathing is important: inhalants help here.

HANGOVER

☞ Drink plenty of water to rehydrate the system.

☞ Ginger and chamomile tea with a good squeeze of lemon juice and a teaspoon of honey will relieve nausea and headache.

☞ Prevention is always best – drink 2–3 glasses of fruit juice and water before bed if you have had more alcohol than usual.

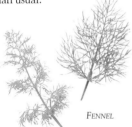

FENNEL

INDIGESTION

☞ Drink peppermint or fennel tea after meals or when feeling full and suffering from gas.

☞ Improve the general tone of the digestive tract with bitter laxative herbs such as dandelion, gentian, and wormwood, taken 20 minutes before food.

☞ A cold stomach can be warmed with the addition of 3 cardamom pods, or a pinch of ginger or cayenne.

ACID INDIGESTION AND HEARTBURN

☞ Avoid rushed and late meals, excessive alcohol, fatty and strongly spiced foods.

☞ Take time to chew fully.

☞ Slippery elm drinks or tablets before meals soothe the stomach. Drinking meadowsweet tea and chewing licorice sticks reduces acidity.

☞ Add chamomile for stress and comfrey to heal gastritis.

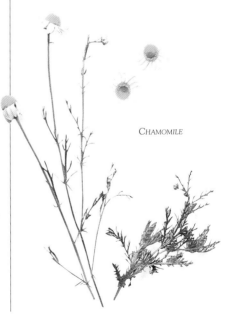

CHAMOMILE

NAUSEA

☞ Ginger tea, or chewing a piece of crystallized ginger, warms the stomach and allays cold nausea.

☞ This can be used for travel sickness or in pregnancy.

☞ Persistent nausea could be a sign of liver problems: seek advice and take dandelion root coffee or decoction.

CONSTIPATION

☞ Poor diet, sedentary lifestyle, and inner stress can all contribute to a sluggish system.

☞ Natural laxatives such as prunes, figs, and fruit juices, together with the natural fiber found in brown rice and vegetables should help. Drink plenty of liquid.

☞ Dock tea and digestive bitters will help improve the tone of the whole alimentary tract.

DIARRHEA

☞ For acute diarrhea, take a gentle laxative such as dock to clear the system.

☞ A few drops of myrrh tincture in water clears many infections.

☞ For chronic and nervous diarrhea use chamomile or marigold mixed with a soothing, astringent herb such as raspberry leaf.

☞ Carrot juice or soup is very helpful, especially for infants.

ANEMIA

☞ Ensure a varied diet and eat regular meals.

☞ Take nettle tea, nettle soup, or eat the young green tops as spinach.

☞ Foods rich in iron, such as spinach, molasses, and apricots, should be added to the diet.

☞ Chinese angelica is traditional for female anemia.

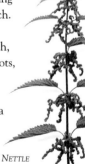

NETTLE

CRAMP

☞ Persistent cramp may be due to mineral deficiencies.

☞ Improve general circulation with hawthorn or rosemary teas. Cramp bark is specific for

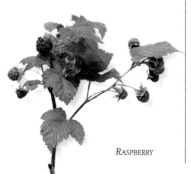

RASPBERRY

stopping attacks: keep some of
the tincture in the house and
take 2–3 teaspoons when it
is needed.

CHILBLAINS

☞ Improve the general
circulation of the body by
taking rosemary tea with a
pinch of cayenne.

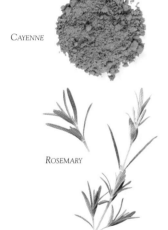

CAYENNE

ROSEMARY

☞ Rub a hot oil, made with
cayenne, pepper, or mustard,
over the chilblain.
☞ Do not apply if the skin is
broken; use marigold ointment
instead. Keep the feet warm at
night or wear bedsocks.

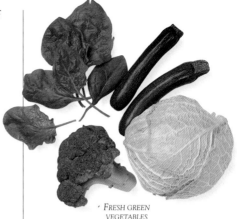

*FRESH GREEN
VEGETABLES*

GOUT

☞ A good diet is the key. Eat
plenty of fresh green vegetables
and avoid high-protein foods
such as red meat and seafood.
☞ Drink plenty of water
and cleansing teas such as
celery seed.
☞ Bring down the acute
inflammation with a compress
of crushed cabbage leaf.

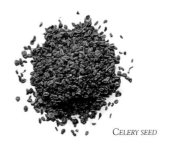

CELERY SEED

VARICOSE VEINS

☞ Avoid standing, sitting, or crossing the legs for long periods. Improve the circulation and muscle tone in the legs with simple toe-clenching and relaxing exercises, and regular short walks.

☞ A cool compress of witch hazel, marigold, or chamomile will help. Drink yarrow tea.

HEMORRHOIDS

☞ Pile wort, or lesser celandine, is specific. Make an ointment in the spring for future use.

☞ Crushed chickweed, or a compress of marigold or chamomile tea, will reduce heat and itching.

☞ Clear congestion in the area with a good diet and teas of bitter herbs such as dock or dandelion root.

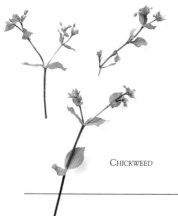

CHICKWEED

ARTERIOSCLEROSIS
(Hardening of the arteries)

☞ Along with stress, this is a major cause of high blood-pressure. Arteriosclerosis is prevented by regular exercise and plenty of garlic in the diet.

☞ Stop smoking, as it makes the symptoms worse.

☞ Take regular herbal teas using hawthorn, horsetail, or linden flowers.

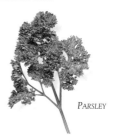

PARSLEY

PERIOD PROBLEMS

☞ As a preventative against cramping pains, drink marigold and raspberry leaf tea on a regular basis.

☞ Cramp bark and ginger tea to relieve attacks.

☞ Agnus castus tea or tablets balances hormones and relieves PMS. Evening primrose oil and sage tea may be helpful for congested breasts.

☞ Drink parsley tea for water retention.

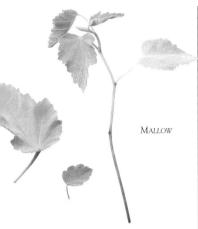

MALLOW

Avoid foods which make the condition worse such as yeast, bread, cheese, and sugar.

Take live bio-yoghurt and marigold tea regularly.

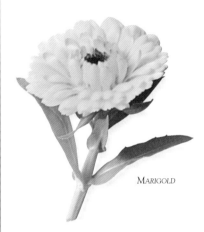

MARIGOLD

CYSTITIS

Drink plenty of water as a preventative.

A teaspoon of lemon juice or sodium bicarbonate in water often relieves an attack.

Herb teas are very effective: they should include a diuretic, such as dandelion leaves, a urinary antiseptic, such as thyme or cranberries, and a soothing herb such as mallow or barley water.

THRUSH

Thyme, myrrh, and sage as a mouthwash or douche.

St. John's wort tincture as a wash and mouthwash.

Add 15 drops of tea tree essential oil to the bath.

ARTHRITIS AND RHEUMATISM

Liniment, a mixture of tincture and oil, makes a good rub.

Juniper tincture and comfrey-infused oil is useful.

Use a cabbage-leaf compress for hot swollen joints.

Parsley, celery seed tea, and dandelion coffee will help with elimination.

Willow bark decoction will help with inflammation.

Glossary

MANY OF THE TERMS *used in this book will be familiar; others may be new to you. All are essential to an understanding of the practice of herbalism.*

ALTERATIVE
Corrects disordered bodily functions

ANALGESIC
Relieves pain

ANTI-EMETIC
Settles the stomach and prevents sickness

ANTI-INFLAMMATORY
Reduces inflammations

ANTISPASMODIC
Alleviates spasms and cramp

ASTRINGENT
Drying

CARMINATIVE
Relaxes the stomach and reduces gas

DECONGESTANT
Relieves congestion

DEMULCENT
Soothes irritation

DIAPHORETIC
Induces sweating

DIURETIC
Promotes urination

EXPECTORANT
Helps expel mucus from the lungs

FEBRIFUGAL
Relieves fever and lowers temperature

LYMPHATIC DEOBSTRUCTANT
Clears swollen lymph nodes, particularly in chronic infection

NERVINE
Strengthens and builds up the nerves

SEDATIVE
Calms the nerves

STIMULANT
Increases activity

STYPTIC
Stems blood flow

TONIC
Strengthens an organ, system, or the whole person

VERMIFUGAL
Kills worms

Further reading

THE COMPLETE ILLUSTRATED
HOLISTIC HERBAL, by *David Hoffman*
(Element Books, 1996)

HERBAL REMEDIES: A PRACTICAL
BEGINNER'S GUIDE TO MAKING
EFFECTIVE REMEDIES IN THE KITCHEN,
by *Christopher Hedley and Non Shaw*
(Parragon, 1996)

THE HERB SOCIETY'S COMPLETE
MEDICINAL HERBAL by *Penny Ody*
(Dorling Kindersley, 1993)

Useful addresses

*For general information on
all aspects of herbs and herbalism:*

The Australian Herb Society
PO Box 110
Mapleton 4560
Australia

The Herb Quarterly
Box 548 MH,
Boiling Springs
PA 17007 USA

The Herb Society
134 Buckingham Palace Road
London SW1W 9SA
UK

*If seeking advice always consult a
qualified practitioner who belongs to a
reputable professional body. The letters
after a name are not the only guide,
word of mouth and personal
recommendations are also important.
The following organizations keep lists
of registered and qualified herbal
practitioners:*

The American Herbalists' Guild
PO Box 1683
Soquel
CA 95073
USA

**The General Council and
Register of Consultant Herbalists**
18 Sussex Square
Brighton
BN2 5AA
UK

**The National Herbalist
Association of Australia**
PO Box 65
Kingsgrove
NSW 2208
Australia

**The National Institute
of Medical Herbalists**
56 Longbrook Street
Exeter
Devon
EX4 6AH
UK